An I of Madness
A diary of a madman. 2011-2017

Josh Alfred

My Early Stages:

I was born 1989, Feb. 27th named Joshua Alfred Washburn. They reported me as brain damaged at birth, but I showed no signs of brain disparity till much later.

Before my symptoms went full blown, emerged and took control, I was young child, home-schooled, and cloistered away from the outside world. I believe it was about 8 years of age, when I started doing home-schooling, and just after then when I would infrequently hear others thoughts. It was a phenomena my therapist would later call a delusion and hallucination, primordial to the full blown mental illness of schizophrenia.

I remember days when I and my brother would try to read each other's minds. My brother could do it too, so I thought it was real. We would probably play that game once or twice every year, too caught up in religion and television to really think outside the box. I remember the first time we did it, and I was thinking "tiger". After about five guesses or so, he thought tiger. It could have been these experiences that would later lead to a stronger telepathic "delusion".

It was the beginning of 2011. I had been laid off nearly a year and a half ago, and couldn't find any work with my meager qualifications. There was no moving out to a new community with more available work opportunities. I was stuck in a rut, receiving half my previous income in unemployment.

My views of the world had changed dramatically in the last year. I had merged with spiritual theoretics. I suddenly understood ideas that were esoteric in nature and that redefined how I thought about reality. I had just finished my book "The Spiritual Cosmos and the Destinies of Humanoids." It included how to open up Chakras. I would later update it after an experience with, what it called itself, an "alien" voice. It was just after I had published this book, along with a new understanding of time and self, a philosophy, that my mind started to go "crazy".

It was a day after my birthday, in February, I was listening to some incredible trance music, and I decided to call out to YAWH, (the alien "god') while looking out the window. I had done this before on another date, when I was 16 and I had seen a UFO. This craft, was one on fire, or consumed in fire traveling from one place than returning to its past position. After a few minutes of listening to the music, I felt energy rise from my spine, and into my brain; sensations I had felt before, but not as intense!

Suddenly there appeared in the sky a blue slash of light. I was unable to see anything but this bluish elongated light, in the night sky. I felt a beam enter my eyes, and my neck gave way. I had blacked out for only a moment, my head falling to my chest. I knew something had changed. For the first time I heard the aliens talk to me. In loud masculine voice, coming from the skies I heard, "What makes you think you can select outcomes better than a higher intelligence?"

I immediately crawled over to my notebook, because I could barely walk at the time, and jotted down this message. (I know I have it somewhere among my many notebooks today.) I am not sure if those were the exact words. At the time I wasn't sure if I could come up with an answer. I was fully convinced that an Alien being had asked me a serious question. I fretfully went over my ideas, and realized that maybe this being was telling me, and as my answers were telling me, that my atheism was interrupting a higher plan. My stubborn atheism collapsed, but only for a while.

In a few minutes I recovered my mobility, but I had this pulsing sensation in my brain every few minutes which continued for the next few days. It was coming from the center of my brain and would move down the sides of my neck, later causing neck spasms, where my head would bobble.

Two days after my 22nd birthday, I was suffering from chronic brain spasms. I hadn't slept in two days, insomnia had set in. It was then that I started to have hallucinations and thought there were spirits around me. I started to communicate with the spirits around me, in what I thought was telepathy. Sometimes I could see the spirits. One was a white being glowing red! I convinced myself that spirits were controlling everything, from my thoughts to the thoughts of my family. I started to hear these spirits talking to one another, they were controlling everything. I had a serious case of de-realization and incredible hallucinations, as the materialistic physicians would say.

I reported to the Doctor, went into the ER, with my brain spasm symptoms, traveling down my neck. After waiting in the waiting room for a few minutes, neck bobbling, the Doctor called me back. He checked me over and said I must have strained some muscles. He gave me some pain reliever, but I wasn't in pain. The pulsations continued, I didn't go to the doctors again for a couple of days, and hardly got any sleep.

During that time, on one day, I went to the store with my brother. Here I fell faint in a few minutes. Everyone was looking at me. I was severely pale and my eye-lids were a reddish pink. I had hardly been out of the house in more than a year.

The next night, it was around 10pm. I was sitting on the sofa and I had my first "euphoric episode." I couldn't move. The "gates of heaven" were opening up to me. I heard my dead father whisper something, and felt his presence next to me. I saw an angel, and all around me glowed gold, platinum, and purple. It was if I was seeing a world on top of this world. I was filled with extreme bliss, and almost started crying. The storm calmed, my mind stopped hallucinating. I can't remember everything I saw that night, nor a lot of what I saw the rest of the year.

That night, after the episode, I realized I couldn't walk ten feet without falling to the ground! Was I becoming paralyzed? It was time to go the emergency room, again. The emergency squad came and carried me out of the apartment. It was a cold winter's night and I ended up shaking from the chill.

Soon, I was in a hospital bed. I started to slip into an unconscious state, but I knew I had to stay awake to find out what was going on with me. I couldn't walk. I felt dizzy, my heart rate started to drop significantly. For awhile I would play with my hands in front of my face, and my heart rate would increase. I found stimulation to keep my mind awake. I decided to tie the shirt I had worn in around my head. I did, suddenly I could walk again. Soon it didn't work for me anymore, and again I collapsed drifting into unconsciousness, heart rate slowing.

My fear had increased, and I could feel panic whenever some one walked into the room. I was thinking "please don't read their minds." About three hours later, I had drifted into a lower conscious state, hypnagogic. It was if I was in a trance. The psychologist walked in. At this time I thought I was hearing the inner voices of everyone around me. I could hear the voices in specific tones, that matched how the people would speak. I was in the lower state of consciousness, when the Doctor some how got me to answer what was I seeing and what was I hearing. Apparently she concluded that I was a psychotic! The nurse came in and gave me some pills, and with them my conscious mind returned.

I was being rolled into the mental health facility at the hospital, out of my mind. I looked at the nurse sitting in the hall-way in front of a door-way. I was convinced that I had been brought to a place where people that heard ghost and were telepathic were brought. I looked at the nurse, and I believed that she was sitting there hearing and seeing ghosts. I didn't think she was a nurse, but some kind of government official who had the same powers that I had.

The nurses would walk up to me, and some of them I would see spirits following them. When they asked me questions, I thought they could read my mind, so I was especially careful about what I thought. People walked by me, pacing the halls. I could hear them, as I stared at them as they walked by. I thought about jumping out the window when they brought me into a room with another man, an older man. He was awake and laying still, with his hand above his eyes. The nurses gave me a decision, I could stay in this room or move to where I was alone. It was tough decision, especially since my mind had gone crazy, and I hadn't slept much in about a week.

I walked over to the man, and said "Hello". I heard his inner voice, in the sound of an old man, and the sound of his voice that I would hear later. It asked, "Are you God?" I thought rhetorically, "What isn't, what is?" We thought a few more things, but then I decided that since he wasn't speaking to me out-loud, and since I was experiencing thought broadcasting that it would be better for me to have my own room. I later found out, that him and another man were suffering from the same kind of mental phenomena as I. One of the men would hide behind a pillar and sit behind just to stop the voices. Eventually, I found myself in that chair, after he left.

When I was first in there, that white walled room, 11x6, I was literally driving my self deeper into insanity. I started to see beings, that I thought were astral projections of the people in the hospital. They had static like bodies. If you took the static off a television with no input signals and reduced it by 50%, and than got it to float around you and float through walls that was about what I was seeing.

The first day I woke up, I swore I was having a stroke from the drugs I had taken. My mouth curved to the side, and I could barely talk or scream. The pulsating was so extreme and wouldn't leave till the next day. No one cared. I couldn't talk. I collapsed. The stroking stopped, and I went to lay down.

I remember looking outside the window and seeing the coal plant nearby, casting fumes into the air. I thought that the nurses were government officials and that they had something to do with global warming. Looking back at it all, it makes me think, makes me wonder how my brain could loss a grip on reality so tragically.

I couldn't escape the voices, they just kept on talking and talking. I was hearing the most I ever did at that time. I started taking pills. They decided to change the pills to Lunesta, a generic anti-psychotic. This lead me into a world of madness. After taking the pill, I started punching walls, swimming on the floor, and screaming out Jim Carey quotes. Everything was green, like the mask, the grinch, the riddler. My face muscles started to feel like they were falling off. The nurses sat me down, and quickly gave me a sleeping pill that almost knocked me out before I could get back to the room.

A week had passed and I was slowly emerging from the chaos of the voices, back into a world where there was a single voice in my head. I would sit in the TV lounge, and swear I was picking up this man's voice. I started to reality test. If I was hearing "you" and were hearing me, "do x." The man sitting across from me had the same thing I had. Once he did what I thought him to do. My later visit to the hospital also brought into contact with a man who "coughed" and laughed after I broadcasted "cough if you can hear me".

The first man kept transmitting thoughts such as "its the same things whales can do. It's just sonar. Your thoughts are bouncing off the walls, like every other frequency." There was more, but I can't remember it. I stopped hallucinating visually, but I was still having auditory hallucinations. That was my first time in. I would revisit two more times, to date.

I don't remember much else about my first stay there. I remember thinking I heard one of the nurses think, "If we were in the wild I'd kill you." A thought that came with derisive look on her face, when she was trying to communicate with me.

These hallucinations weren't just an altered state of consciousness, they were also a cause for fear and distress, and would be for some time.

Finally, my symptoms had decreased to a point where the doctors thought I could go home. It was about a week and half. At home, that first month, I had another euphoric experience, about the same things happened. I was convinced that what I was hearing was "spirit", and that they had something to do with human destiny. I started to read the Bible, probably not the best thing to do, but it has been shown the schizophrenics suddenly turn religious. I was looking for answers, rather than wanting to convert. I read revelations mostly, because therein it tells of how Jesus and God both come to earth in "thrones" and "clouds" which might be interpreted as space-crafts.

I read the part where it says, angels are out in front of the Churches and are awaiting Christ's return. It made me imagine so vividly that I was in some kind of game, a simulation of sorts, where in the view from heaven, there were just these characters, and spiritual beings interacting with one another. It was much like thinking of SIMS or the game Diablo, and I guess that's probably where those ideas came from.

Eventually I put down the Bible, and stopped reading it all together. There were no tangible answers, just verses that construed some unbelievable story. I can't remember any vivid visual hallucinations or any meaningful voices that I was hearing during the first two months. I would go into an "aphasia episode" almost every day, where all I could hear were the voices, and I wasn't sure what people were saying to me.

When I moved out of that apartment, and into a larger one, the voices I was hearing from the upstairs neighbors had vanished, and I felt a reduction of stress. I had stopped taking Risperdal, and strated on Sapharis (after the first few months).

At first my psychotic attacks, where the voices would overcome my voice that I know as "my internal voice", would happen only on Sunday. I remember reading Revelations, and thinking of John of Patmos experiences. He might have been just as psychotic as I was. Eventually, I would have an attack every night.

Sapharis reduced the psychotic and aphasia attacks I was having to 2-3 per week, but for me it was still tormenting getting through every day. I would probably hear 5hr or more of voices, and fond clarity some days more than others.

I remember the night when I started to talk to an alien being. I could hear my spirit guide telling me that she was communicating with this being and through her I would be talking. It was then that I added more onto my book about the possibility of the spirit in the universe. I had been told, that there were universes other than ours, where beings existed that had proliferated most if not all of their universe. Basically, filled with life everywhere. It said, that our universe was like this, and one could think of it in terms of "percent complete." I don't remember much more of the message, but I remember talking (telepathically) for an hour or so.

All through the months I was convinced that I was talking to beings using thought alone.

One day the voices, and my mind suddenly turned against the world. As my therapist described it, "did you feel a sense of evil overcome you?" As I answered, "yes." I couldn't stop repeating threats, they just came out. I wasn't angry, or frustrated at all, something other than what I knew as the happy me, the normal me, had been possessed by a foreign consciousness.

I ended up being brought into the ward handcuffed. I hadn't hurt anyone, my mind was simply gone and I just kept repeating the same threats over and over again, in a very quiet and fast voice. That was my second visit to the hospital. I believe that's when they started me on the new drug (Sapharis).

I remember getting home and being so much more clear of thought. I don't remember anything significant happening that second visit.

I was on that pill for many months, and finally of February this year, I broke down again. The pill stopped working.

Some of my experiences before the third visit to the hospital were of alien kind. I would see multiple aliens in what I would call my conscious field. One after another, come and go. Some would make this squeaking noise and than my spirit guide (the female voice that I heard most of the time would translate). It is an experience much like someone reports after taking hallucinogenic drugs.

I tried astral traveling, and went to a world were a being flew in glowing orb space-crafts, in sparkling skies filled with some kind of chemical dust. I remember hovering over my body, and seeing myself, much like depicted in Alex Grey's artwork. The aliens that I would see were sometimes robots. One was amazing, and I might use it as a pro-type for building a robot in the future.

I remember one night sitting out on the porch with my computer. This man's voice suddenly appeared. I felt him standing outside the window (closed in porch). You talk about the wiles. There's nothing like thinking that an invisible being is standing and talking in front of you. I don't remember what the man said, but I rushed off the porch and told my spirit guide, "I will have nothing to do with talking to the dead."

One night, the weirdest and most amazing experience I have ever had, took place. I was lying down in bed. First I saw this woman, wearing a short dress. She was all gray, and see-through, ethereal. She was dancing around me, pulling up some kind of rope from around my body. Eventually, she flew upward into the sky. From my forehead I could see this gray rope going up to the skies. I have thought about it a lot, but probably never know what it was for sure. I remember putting my hand through the rope and watching it as organized smoke go out of place and back into place. After this a large male angel appeared next to me.

I looked over and I could see the hem of his clock, and I could feel this energy coming from him. He/she (androgynous) was standing nine-feet tall. He said something, but I can't remember it, nor did I document it, being so late at night. The last thing I saw that was something I would again, just recently but not from a spirit world. A teleportation portal here an image (there are many) and a video:

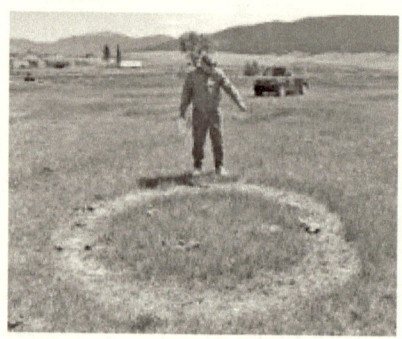

The teleportation portal was opened vertically not horizontally as in this (horizontal) footage>. This may be a fake, but to get a visual of what I saw this is perfect rendition.

I don't know what came through it, but something leaped through the door frame were it appeared out toward my bed.

Off my pills, I will usually see faces, aliens, robots, angels, or hear the voices of some

being trying to talk to me, as well spirals
that are just as ethereal as these beings. They
remind me of worm-holes in a way.

I also remember seeing this alien with a
huge head, about 2 1/2 feet in diameter. It
kept saying, "Eternal form and function." I
called my therapist that day, and he said to
wait it out. I did. I told him what the Alien
was saying to me on my next appointment,
through my spirit guide. He was just
stunned, having no other response. Perhaps,
I made him think of Platonism.

I remember two other alien encounters. I
was lying in bed, and felt like I was asleep
and paralyzed. An alien appeared above me,
glowing green, a head much like an oval
vase turned upside down. It said something
like, "I am here to fix you." I felt my brain
twitching, like neurons were being clipped. I
was bothered, and wanted to wake up. I
don't remember exactly what happened, but
I remember seeing the same thing twice in
that night, the alien above, moving its
fingers as my brain was tickled.

Another occurrence that happened three times, I could see this alien with a large head, made of gray, but when it expanded itself towards me it would glow yellow. I felt immense sense of love coming from it, not an emotional intensity I would feel from any other being. It had equanimity about it, yet I could feel radiation of emotion coming from its core when it expanded towards me.

My next serious attack was just a few months ago. I started saying random things, and didn't know what was going on. I started to hear this woman basically threaten me, and she would try to calm me down sometimes by saying, "Mushroom cloud" just get way from the insanity I was hearing. It didn't seem to calm me much at all, because it made me think of an atomic bomb. This time too, I was too fucked out of my mind to write anything down. I started repeating "Angels, angels, angels, angels" about 80 times per minute and my eyes would roll back into my head. I ended up in the hospital for a third time.

This time in the hospital my heart rate went up to 200bpm every few minutes, and I couldn't breathe. I had stopped repeating angels after being in the hospital for a few minutes. They gave me oxygen fifteen minutes in. I started to see a huge body in front of me. It would take up most of my conscious field. It would get out of its a chair and back into it, and would torture me with its thoughts.

The doctor came in, and just before I had seen an alien, with an oval head blue and white head, come into my conscious field than disappear. The doctor asked me what I was seeing. I told her Aliens, I started seeing four that wouldn't leave. Finally they got me some meds that calmed me down, and it was back into the ward.

Finally after this visit they put me on a drug that has been working great for me, Seraquil.

At first I would hear voices 2 hrs a day, and have a single attack in a week. Now, as of September 18th 2012, I rarely hear voices. I recently moved again, into an A-frame. The other night, I had hallucinations of spiders twice. I also awoke to see a boy standing outside my door. Looking straight ahead. He was wearing a tank top and was about four feet tall, possibly Hispanic. I looked at him, then he noticed I was looking and hid behind the door frame, with his head and eyes peeking in at me. I looked backed, gazing at him, and then he was gone.

I stared at the place he was in, telling my self it was all just a hallucination. I still have questions though, why spiders, aliens, angels, an unreal boy, a man with a presence? I don't know, we don't know. Nor do I know if my mind is psychic or imbalanced, or if I am a psychic mind gone mad. I have seen lots of positive proof that has shown some of things I have undergone and still undergo (thought broadcasting). One of the shows that gets at these phenomena being extra-natural is "Fifth Dimension". I also have told the future a couple of times, after hearing it from a spirit guide. This reminds of the abilities of the "psychic twins" who accurately predicted the 9/11 attack, even warning us of it.

I live as though I am crazy, but am skeptical about whether or not I am medium. In other cultures, schizophrenics are called Shamans. In our culture we are called the insane, given some money to hardly live off of, waiting to recover.

Sometimes I want to go off my pills, just to see this altered world that is hidden from a "healthy" consciousness. Then I remember what my doctor say, going off your meds can reverse the effects of the drugs. So I know that to do what is best for me, I must stop thinking of such things, and move on with what is culture normality.

I have recovered on new pills. The only real problem with my mind I have these days in thought-broadcasting. Even sometimes I will have a scientifically uncategorized type of thought broadcasting, looking at some one from the past, and hearing their voice just as if they would say it. I can live and go on functioning in society with my voices being as low as they are now. I have a plan for myself, and if my mind doesn't want to do it, if I fall sick again, then again I will pick myself up, and try to recover.

If this story interested you or you have had similar experiences, feel free to share. I am willing to detail any my experiences as much as possible.

As of October 15th, my voices came back for a weeks and were constantly on my case, some giving me insight, some just commentary. A couple weeks ago, I remember my heart rate increasing. I had a vision that night, of a 2d torus pattern with an eye in the middle, colors all around it. My low blood pressure mixed with potassiums (bananas), cause my heart to race, as the correlation has appeared before. Now I know if I just want a trip, all I have to do is eat a few bananas, or have something with high potassium, and my heart rate will go up, and I will see things. It may come with risks, but its better than going off meds to "hear the voices clearly"'.

During these weeks I would try to answer
questions on online forum using the voices
as guidance, at night, when they were really
active. I think I shared insight and generated
some myself.

On another note, since I have moved, my
spirit guide has seemingly changed. Instead
of a rather high-pitched female voice, I hear
the voice of soothing female. After
potassium intake her voice is loud and clear,
coming from around me. I haven't noted
what she was saying yet, but I will try to
remember to write some things down, if I do
return to that state.

Nov 15th/2011

Not much has happened in the last month. I
was planing to go back to school, but I don't
think it going to happen till after Jan.

One experience that I did have that has
frightened me a bit, was one night I was
sleeping looking towards my doorway.
There appeared a black figure. It teleported
from one position to the next till it was

standing next to my bed, and that's when I saw her. A woman draped in white, even covering her head. All that I could see was her gray hair, bangs covering her eyes. She was white, but with tan. I wouldn't have been as frightened but I saw here twice.

The other night, I saw a plasma body, not with much form, standing next to my bed on the other side, but I refused to look at it for longer than a second. I know my mind might be fabricating these things itself. It has made me think and question, "why is imagination usually scattered, while these visions are so clear and concrete at times?" Even the aliens I have seen, they are much like looking a real thing but existing in another field. These experiences are either of another function of mind or paranormal activity.

I haven't been out much, so haven't had that many experiences with TB. I did experience it a couple times, while watching television, as I have been experiencing for awhile. Nothing of importance.

I remember a time when I first came down with the disease. I was seeing people, and I could see their foreheads, and inside them glowing a bright yellow light. They also had horns and a halo. This happened for about two days, and than I saw a crop circle. It was at this time I was concluding that man is somehow a mix between angel and demon, but it just seems so far-fetched now that I don't see these properties on a regular basis. This symptom? Totally awesome! Some people had far larger glowing inside their head, and it would take me back. Others I could see the horns on them more than then their other attributes.

11/26/12

Last night a heard an aliens voice, say one of my pseduo-names "Juefawn." It appeared for a few seconds, and pointed at me. It was yellow gold, with a shine to its skin. Its eyes were golden with dark pupils. The eyes were smaller than the size of a baseball, not almond, but circular; distinctive facial features. Brains mostly set like ours, skull more round.

6/1/2014

It has been about six months since things have changed for me. I used to hear differing consistent voices. I used to hear two females and one male. I had given them names. It was Micheal and The Feminine. These consistent voices existed about five to six months ago. Now Micheal has been replaced. I started to use a mental diagram of the voices. This was of three points, so I formed it into a triangle, and called each voice a number.

Eventually this diagram wasn't sufficient. After this Micheal seemed to disappear. I started hearing more than three consistent voices. I no longer hear Micheal, and sometimes ask myself where his voice went, even though there is obviously no realistic answer to this question for me. I still use the triangle diagram, 1 male, 2 feminine (like mother's voice) 3 feminine. However, 1 is no longer the same male voice that I heard normally.

Among these voices there is the male that mostly says, "I don't care." This has become a consistent thought pattern in his voice. He says other things, but I do not keep track of them. I think his psychic energy might be defined as "assisting in diminishing about my own thoughts/cares. Another voices says "Loser" which seems to have the voice of a girl I used to know, but I can't be sure of this with human memory being so unreliable.

The voice of "I don't care" has come about as a consequence of not putting mental efforts in answering questions online. I seem to realize that my own life is of more relevance and that it takes more mental effort to use my intelligence on social networks opining and scrutinizing. My intelligence has decreased with my lack of use with writing on the net. The computer bolsters my intelligence, and without it I become less aware and less preoccupied with the things of the world. I question to myself, "Will never using the computer again cause me to more or less ill?" Too much seems to be agitating, making my

symptoms worse, to little seems to make my
intelligence less functional.

Health is a priority. Learning what is healthy
and not healthy is difficult to discern. Doing
what makes you healthy is also difficult to
put into action. There both even harder when
your brain is dysfunctional. Once you know
what agitated you or makes you sick you
bare the knowledge of what to do, but
possibly not the will to follow through with
the healthier concept of life.

A set of voices I hear are two which seem to
share opposite psychic energy. I would call
one a pleaser and one the resistor ((7) the
consistent voice). They might have
something to do with my own sexual
energies, but I can't make sense of this. If I
do one thing more than the other, experience
pleasure or not, the two will come out. I am
overstimulated sexually, and there is a
natural resistance to this, which comes
through as the two conflicting voices. I can't
make much sense of this either. It should be
something I bring up with a therapist but I
don't feel sure I can talk about these matters.

I have noticed that my own internal voice, has disappeared. This often leaves me in a stupor of wonder. Among other questions I ask if I will ever get my internal voice back? Its liked be robbed of your own heartbeat. I want to discover if there is something I can do to bring back my own voice.

I have experienced with frequency tones. I wanted to see what would happen upon listening to different frequencies. This lead me to conclude that certain sounds trigger certain voices. I think this means I am experiencing a different type of consciousness, almost like I belong to a different species. Yet I know I am a human being, there is just some differences/abnormalities in genes, brain processing, and environment factors.

Reading Bible = I read the Bible for two weeks. At doing this there were differing voices for this timespan. There was one male voice I remember from the time. This male voice would chant verses, repeating them, but so in-distinctively I could not hear him. I did feel better after reading the Bible, and memorizing some verses, but I don't get the purpose of reading it exactly (since my science doesn't mix well with my religion).

After a few days of not reading the Bible for a few days, if I remember correctly the old voices came back. This occurred after nearly last summer.

(6/2013) As with experimenting with frequency I might attempt to gather information on my own illness by taking part in following through on a religious life. But should this really be the purpose of religion? See how it effects your life?

Dodo brain = This is a name a voice gave me. I think it would mean that because of the brain I have my own genome or branch of offspring who have my disease are destined for extinction. More simply, that I would never survive or be able to function in the wild, or perhaps even society which requires its ill to earn survival through working.

I often notice there are changes in my thought patterns that change voices. This means that over time I will probably experience a change in the voices. The "hack" is the trial of different activities to induce differing mental experience. Though hacks or strategies to change mental experience might exist, I try to remember I cannot cure myself entirely, just that my mind is changeable.

I have gone without seeing a therapist for 6 months or more, and my consciousness is more split. It's a reason to get out of the house and talk to someone. I think this intention is good, good for my mental health.

—

5/4/2014

It has been over a year, where do I start? My mom, brother, and I moved south to North Carolina. We moved there from upstate New York, Here there was a new hospital to visit. I am still visiting the hospital about every six months. I tell myself this time, on this medication, just maybe I will have a full recovery. I have tried about 5 different pills, and this one is working well.

What hallucinations have I had that still are with me today? I still experience thought broadcasting and want to write more about how that confuses me.

I tried being religious. I gave up on being an Author under a delusional state of mind. I also threw away a ring of mine that had sentimental value. I just wanted to start over, and that's what I plan on doing. Out of all the 20 some books and 250 poems I have written there are only a few that survived my trashing binge. I deleted all my books, and promised to God that I wouldn't write another book that didn't serve his purposes. Afterward, I found this way too narrowing. There is hardly any telling what a person can do if they take religion to seriously. That's the truth -- how it's always been. There was something in the Book that changed me. On top of the dogma of the book there was my own self-doubt that contributed to me deleting some of my work. I wanted to start over, and that's what I am deciding to do as of this year. I have run low on book ideas, and still want to go to college for writing and psychology. If only I had degrees my Authoring books might go somewhere, (meaning sell).

The hospital here is insufficient to treat people with psychosis, meaning there is no special mental ward in the area I moved to. I advise that those who are mentally ill think about the location and accommodations the health community has for your disease and treatment. This way you will be able to get the service you need.

I was in the hospital twice last year, or about the same things. I believe it was November when I made my second visit in 2014. That time I had gone in again to the emergency room. I knew now how I would be treated there. Throw a prescription and move on. I didn't get help locally they had to transport me to a different county having a ward there. This time in I had started to hear yelling voices.

Hallucinations: On a drug I had been on for about six months, I started to hear and sense entities. You see the brain isn't well understood. How can a normal brain, normal conscious brain, produce a sense of presence and sharing space with entities – entities that spoke and had different intelligences, having a mind of their own? This is a tough question to answer and I leave it to the experts to deliberate on.

As far as seeing things go, I started seeing these images of Gold, made up of a gold outlines. Later I would see these images at the school I was going to. One image was of an Aztec pyramid. I soon found myself starting at an education program that used the Aztec pyramid on its home page screen. One minute I am sitting in my living room hallucinating the next I am looking at the image at school. That's one case. Others have been in blue, pink, purple only. They vibrate like they are made of static and and vibrant light.

What do I hallucinate? Instead of seeing whole beings glowing there is a light around them, and some kind of spooky translucent glow to the shapes inside the outlines.

Why does this happen? There is obviously something occurring uniquely in my visual cortex. This reminds me of the thought process that takes place in the man named Dan Tammet. He reports to visualize colors in blobs that equal numbers. While his comes with math my comes with voices. I do not hallucinate math symbols and numbers, instead I hallucinate in language. The question arises, do we hallucinate or visualize? There is a fine line between the two. Visualizations can often come with deciding to think something, while hallucinations appear on their own and are not as effected by a mind's decision. I didn't ask for any of this -- something most mentally dysfunctional might say.

Apophenia - I stayed in bed for five days straight. It is the bed of rolling-around-in-your-own-misery, a depressive state. I started to experience apophenia symptoms while in bed. All the marks and patterns started to vibrating in cartoon renditions of thought. If I started thinking about eating noodles I'd see a cartoon eating noodles. If I decided to think of rabbits, I'd see a cartoon version jump up and down. Still the mystery remains do I decide to see these things or do they come up first? Maybe I am right to think I just can't know.

11/12/2015

Recently, I was in the hospital twice within the period of two months. I started to hear voices telling me to kill myself. If you have these symptoms and are asked about them, giving a true answer, you find yourself in a hospital involuntarily committed. This happened to me twice in two months.

The first time I was committed my Doctor was the one to call the police on me and have me detained and brought to the hospital. It had been a year since I was in the hospital with florid symptoms. The second time I walked down the street to the hospital, going there only to receive a particular drug which stops me from shaking uncontrollably. The second time, I was asked if I was having suicidal thoughts, to which I replied, "yes". After my second visit of 18 days in a rehab facility I no longer hear voices. They put me on a new anti-psychotic which seems to be working for now.

My hallucinations now are visual. I will still see the outline of bodies and faces. The outlines are blue or red, shining, flickering, fading in seconds and appearing for seconds.

4/5/2016

Its been six years now and my symptoms have worsened. I didn't used to hallucinate as badly as I do now. Now when I hallucinate I will see images in monotonous colors. For example I will see faces in green, purple, red or yellow. These faces aren't like what you imagine them to be, they are cartoonish and unique. The faces will be in excess of four or five and be spinning, grinning, shouting, grimacing, or open with jagged teeth, horrific in nature. When I look out at the world this is what I will be seeing. When I look into your eyes it is likely that I

am hallucinating images on the space of
your face, most likely the forehead as I
make eye contact difficultly. They linger in
day to day life, but are bad when having a
weekly episode.

My voices now have a poverty of thought to
them, obtrusive and confused. I start
thinking illogically, and I can't seem to form
long coherent thoughts but I am more able to
do so when not having an episode. I have an
episode weekly, and when this happens I'm
subject to voices and visions that occupy the
totality of my mind. I no longer can hold a
train of thought or think of visuals outside of
what I am hallucinating. I lose all control,
the kind you think you have when you go to
think of your next thoughts.

As far as drugs go I am on an oral
medication and an injection. I take zypraxia
and invega. I take ten mgs twice a day and
am injected with 160mg shot every month.
The injection hurts when the needle sticks in
my arm and than I will get a lasting sore on
my arm for a few days afterward.

Right now I suffer from obesity and weigh over 190lbs. I have gained a lot of wait this year so far, and it is mostly noticeable in my stomach region. My belly is large and this is where most of my weight is. I am thinking about doing an exercise routine to lose weight and too cut back on my soda intake.

The only other side-effect I have is drooling, which happens at random times and it is sometimes a laugh. I could be taking meds for this side-effect but I am trying to not be on any meds I don't have to be on.

One thing I do to stop an episode is put my focus onto a game I can play on my tablet or my computer. Not everyone has this luxury but it does work for me.

I have been in an ACT workshop now for a year. It's a group of people assigned to treat you at your home. There are about four people that come to see me and talk to me throughout the month. I don't have a therapist only a counselor who comes to chat with me for a few minutes every week. My psychiatrist will show up every month or so and ask me about my symptoms. They have worsened, and I gather that I am growing tolerant to my medication as I have with all of them. I hardly heard voices at first now I have an episode weekly.

1/20/2017

I went into the ER 4 times in November. I was stricken with psychotic symptoms and aphasia symptoms. They have been present with some increased severity and being recrudescent since sometime in the summer.

What happens is: I lose my center of focus, become intermixed in a chaotic storm of auditory wrestling winds. There is no more center to myself, as I start to repeat my thoughts and what others say. With jostling repetition I lose my coherence.

I see images popping out of patterns on the walls and floors, and sometimes even see them come out of no patterns whatsoever. It's obvious that my visual pattern recognition is somehow and somewhat skewed -- aberrant neurologically.

I hear often perverted, homicidal, suicidal voices, male and female. The same I have been hearing for years. While in the hospital these voices seem to magnify in quantity, and often the familiars become dormant.

Right now as far as medication I have been prescribed a "benzo" which is very multi-usable in treatment of mania, anxiety, agitation, and for me aphasia and psychotic symptoms.

After taking a very small as-needed-dosage of the drug my symptoms become mostly intangible. I still can't hear my inner voice very clearly, but my clarity is always improved. Thanks to this regimen I have evade any emergency medical treatment.

You may ask yourself why is this condition of episodes an emergency event? It is really the fright that makes me feel as though I am in danger, and I do most often think of myself as more dangerous when I am florid.

More life-related: I have moved twice, From a 4 bdrm home, to a 1 bdrm, to a 2 bdrm. It has really been my mom that has wanted to move and I have stayed with her. I became a victim of her control. Her decisions to move have not been highly rational considering the job opportunities where we live now are almost naught.

I wanted to go back to work here, but it doesn't appear to be fortuitous. I also want to finish schooling but this too seems like chasing a rabbit out of its cage. I will reach my egoic ideals eventually, but for now I am in stagnation.

———

When watching people discuss things, when people engage, I am faced with degrees of confusion (By confusion here I mean a disturbance of one's focus.). These are : 1) body language, 2) what the person is saying, 3) who their voice is directed to while voices go on inside my head.

The body language, such as facial expressions stands out and seems to inform me.

What the person is saying is more relevant than their gestures, most times.

Who the voices are directed to is often simple, but not when in groups. Here I get confused of who is being talked to.

Lastly, the voices I am hearing are in some degree like most voices in the head, they are trying to be said.

———

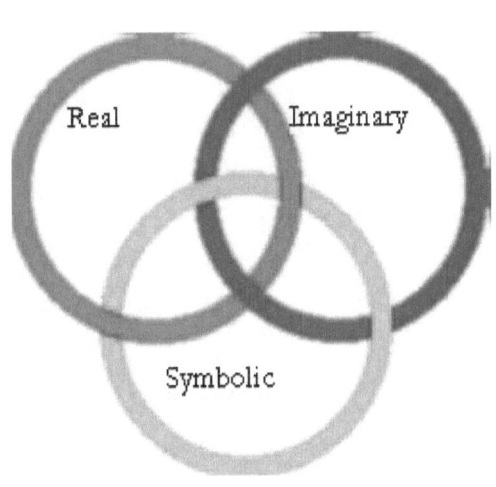

Above we a have logical-visual aid (Borromean Knnot) to represent how a normal psyche's dynamics are interwined. In psychosis you get a singular collection within the triad, or more easy to envision a total convergence. This is a Lacan psychodynamic representation, and in regards schizophrenic psychosis accurately represents the "hijacking of the imagination and the word" in my experiences.